Copyright ©

All rights reserved. No part of this publication may be reproduced, distributed, or transmitted in any form or by any means, including photocopying, recording, or other electronic or mechanical methods, without the prior written permission of the publisher, except in the case of brief quotations embodied in critical reviews and certain other noncommercial uses permitted by copyright law.

Contents

Understanding Candida: Causes, Symptoms, and Effects

Candida overgrowth is a common health concern that affects many individuals worldwide. Candida is a type of yeast that naturally exists in our bodies, primarily in the gastrointestinal tract. Under normal circumstances, the presence of candida is balanced by beneficial bacteria and other microorganisms. However, certain factors can disrupt this balance, leading to an overgrowth of candida and causing various health issues.

Causes of Candida Overgrowth:

Several factors can contribute to the development of candida overgrowth. These include:

Antibiotic Use: Antibiotics, while effective in fighting bacterial infections, can also kill beneficial bacteria in the gut. This disruption in the gut microbiome can allow candida to multiply and cause an overgrowth.

Weakened Immune System: A compromised immune system, whether due to chronic illnesses, stress, or poor nutrition, can make individuals more susceptible to candida overgrowth.

Diet High in Sugar and Processed Foods: Candida feeds on sugar and processed carbohydrates, so a diet rich in these foods can contribute to candida overgrowth.

Hormonal Changes: Hormonal fluctuations, such as those occurring during pregnancy, menopause, or the use of hormonal birth control, can create an environment favorable for candida overgrowth.

Chronic Stress: Prolonged periods of stress can weaken the immune system and disrupt the balance of microorganisms in the body, potentially leading to candida overgrowth.

Symptoms of Candida Overgrowth: Candida overgrowth can manifest in various ways, and the symptoms may vary from person to person. Common symptoms include:

Digestive Issues: These can include bloating, gas, diarrhea, constipation, and abdominal pain.

Recurrent Yeast Infections: Candida overgrowth can cause frequent vaginal yeast infections in women, as well as oral thrush.

Fatigue and Low Energy: Individuals with candida overgrowth often experience persistent fatigue, even after getting enough sleep.

Brain Fog and Poor Concentration: Candida can produce toxins that affect cognitive function, leading to difficulties with focus, memory, and mental clarity.

Skin and Nail Infections: Candida can cause fungal infections on the skin, such as athlete's foot or fungal nail infections.

Effects of Candida Overgrowth: If left untreated, candida overgrowth can have a significant impact on overall health and well-being. Some potential effects include:

Nutrient Malabsorption: Candida overgrowth can impair the absorption of essential nutrients, leading to deficiencies and related health issues.

Weakened Immune System: Candida overgrowth can compromise the immune system, making individuals more susceptible to other infections and illnesses.

Inflammation and Allergies: The presence of candida can trigger an inflammatory response in the body, leading to allergies and other immune-related reactions.

Disruption of Gut Health: Candida overgrowth disrupts the balance of microorganisms in the gut, which can negatively affect digestion, nutrient absorption, and overall gut health.

Chronic Health Conditions: There is evidence linking candida overgrowth to conditions such as irritable bowel syndrome (IBS), fibromyalgia, chronic fatigue syndrome, and autoimmune diseases.

Candida Diet Basics: Getting Started

What is the Candida Diet?

The candida diet is a therapeutic approach aimed at reducing candida overgrowth by eliminating foods that nourish candida and promoting those that support a healthy gut environment. The diet focuses on removing foods high in sugar, refined carbohydrates, and yeast, as these are the primary fuel sources for candida.

Why Follow the Candida Diet?

Following the candida diet can help restore the balance of microorganisms in the gut and alleviate the symptoms associated with candida overgrowth. By eliminating candida-promoting foods and incorporating nutrient-dense, anti-inflammatory foods, individuals can support their immune system, reduce inflammation, and create an environment that discourages candida growth.

Foods to Avoid on the Candida Diet:

To effectively combat candida overgrowth, it is essential to avoid or minimize certain foods that can contribute to its growth. These include:

Sugar and Artificial Sweeteners: This includes refined sugar, honey, maple syrup, agave nectar, and artificial sweeteners like aspartame and sucralose.

Refined Carbohydrates: White bread, pasta, pastries, and processed cereals should be avoided, as they can quickly break down into sugar and fuel candida growth.

Yeast-Containing Foods: Foods made with yeast, such as bread, rolls, and baked goods, should be eliminated, as yeast can contribute to candida overgrowth.

Alcohol: Alcohol is high in sugar and can disrupt the balance of gut microorganisms, making it important to avoid during the candida diet.

Moldy Foods: Moldy or fungi-contaminated foods, including moldy cheeses, peanuts, and dried fruits, should be avoided, as they can exacerbate candida symptoms.

2.4 Foods to Include on the Candida Diet: The candida diet emphasizes nutrient-dense, anti-inflammatory foods that support gut health and help combat candida overgrowth. Foods to include on the candida diet include:

Non-Starchy Vegetables: Leafy greens, cruciferous vegetables, asparagus, zucchini, and cucumber are excellent choices as they provide essential nutrients and fiber.

Lean Proteins: Opt for sources like fish, poultry, eggs, and legumes, as they are rich in protein and support healthy digestion.

Healthy Fats: Avocado, coconut oil, olive oil, and nuts and seeds are healthy sources of fats that can help reduce inflammation and provide sustained energy.

Fermented Foods: Incorporate fermented foods like sauerkraut, kimchi, kefir, and yogurt (unsweetened and dairy-free) into your diet to promote a healthy gut microbiome.

Antifungal Herbs and Spices: Garlic, oregano, ginger, turmeric, and cinnamon have antifungal properties and can be included in meals to support candida control.

By following the candida diet guidelines and making appropriate food choices, individuals can create an environment in their bodies that discourages candida overgrowth and promotes overall health and well-being.

What is Candidiasis?

There are many kinds of fungus that live in the human body. One type is called candida. It's a type of yeast that normally lives in small amounts in places like your mouth and belly, or on your skin without causing any problems. But when the environment is right, the yeast can multiply and grow out of control.

The infection it causes is called candidiasis. There are several different types of it. Most can be easily treated with over-the-counter or prescription medications.

Thrush (Oropharyngeal Candidiasis)

When the candida yeast spreads in the mouth and throat, it can cause an infection called thrush. It's most common in newborns, the elderly and people with weakened immune systems. Also more likely to get it are adults who:

Are being treated for cancer

Take medications like corticosteroids and wide-spectrum antibiotics

Wear dentures

Have diabetes

The symptoms include:

White or yellow patches on the tongue, lips, gums, roof of mouth, and inner cheeks

Redness or soreness in the mouth and throat

Cracking at the corners of the mouth

Pain when swallowing, if it spreads to the throat

Thrush is treated with antifungal medicines like nystatin, clotrimazole, and fluconazole. Rinsing the mouth with chlorhexidine (CHX) mouthwash may help prevent infections in people with weakened immune systems.

Genital Yeast Infection (Genital Candidiasis)

Three out of four adult women will get at least one yeast infection during their lifetime. This occurs when too much yeast grows in the vagina. (Men also can get a genital yeast infection, but it's much less common).

A yeast infection typically happens when the balance in the vagina changes. This can be caused by pregnancy, diabetes, use of some medicines, lubricants, or spermicides, or a weakened immune system. Occasionally, the infection can be passed from person to person during sex.

The symptoms include:

- Extreme itchiness in the vagina

- Redness and swelling of the vagina and vulva (the outer part of the female genitals)

- Pain and burning when you pee

- Discomfort during sex

- A thick, white "cottage cheese" discharge from the vagina

- A man with a yeast infection may have an itchy rash on their penis.

Portobello Mushrooms Stuffed with Barley Risotto

INGREDIENTS

- 4 large portobello mushroom caps

- 2 tablespoons extra-virgin olive oil

- Kosher salt and freshly ground black pepper

- 4 cups vegetable or chicken broth

- 2 tablespoons unsalted butter

- 1 sweet onion, chopped

- 3 garlic cloves, minced

- 1 cup barley

- ½ cup white wine

- 4 ounces baby kale or spinach

- 2 teaspoons chopped fresh thyme

- 1 teaspoon chopped fresh rosemary

- ½ cup grated Parmesan cheese, plus more for garnish

- Chopped fresh parsley, for serving

DIRECTIONS

1. Preheat the oven to 375°F. Line a baking sheet with parchment paper. Brush the mushroom caps with the olive oil and season with salt and pepper. Transfer to the baking sheet.

2. In a medium saucepan, heat the broth over medium-low heat. Keep warm over low heat.

3. In another medium pot, melt the butter over medium heat. Add the onion and sauté until translucent, about 5 minutes. Add the garlic and sauté until fragrant, about 1 minute more.

4. Add the barley and cook for 45 seconds, stirring constantly. Add the white wine and bring

to a simmer; stir until the wine is mostly absorbed by the grains.

5. Begin adding the broth in batches, 1 to 2 ladles full at a time. Stir the barley and broth frequently, allowing it to simmer vigorously. When the barley has absorbed almost all the broth, add another 1 to 2 ladles full and continue to stir until all the broth is absorbed. Continue until all of the broth is used and the barley is tender (if needed, use water to complete cooking). The process will take about 30 to 40 minutes.

6. Meanwhile, roast the mushrooms until they're just tender, 12 to 15 minutes. When you remove them from the oven, flip them over to allow any excess liquid or oil to drain out.

7. Stir the baby kale or spinach into the risotto until it's wilted. Add the thyme and rosemary; season with salt and pepper. Add the Parmesan and stir vigorously to combine. The risotto should look thick and creamy.

8. To serve, divide the risotto among the mushroom caps. Garnish the risotto with more Parmesan and parsley. Serve immediately.

Lemon-Tahini Salad with Lentils, Beets and Carrots

INGREDIENTS

- 3 small beets, scrubbed

- ¾ cup small green lentils

- Kosher salt

- 3 tablespoons tahini

- 2 tablespoons fresh lemon juice

- 1 teaspoon honey

- Freshly ground pepper

- 1 small onion, finely chopped

- 2 lightly packed cups baby kale

- 1 romaine heart, chopped

- 1½ cups diced carrots

DIRECTIONS

1. Fill a deep skillet with ½ inch water and bring to a simmer over medium heat. Add the beets, cover, and cook until tender, about 20 minutes. Drain and run the beets under cold water to cool. Rub off the skins and then dice.

2. Meanwhile, in a small saucepan, combine the lentils and enough water to cover by 2 inches; bring to a boil over high heat. Cover partially, reduce the heat to medium and simmer until the lentils are tender, 20 to 25 minutes. Season with salt and let stand 5 minutes, then drain off any excess water.

3. In a large bowl, whisk together the tahini, lemon juice, honey and 2 tablespoons water; season with salt and pepper. Add the onion and let stand 5 minutes.

4. Add the kale, romaine heart, carrots, beets and lentils; toss to combine and then season with salt and pepper.

Ultra Crispy Baked Potato Wedges

INGREDIENTS

- 2 pounds Russet potatoes (6 smallish or 4 medium), scrubbed clean (I didn't peel mine)

- 3 tablespoons olive oil

- 2 teaspoons garlic powder

- 2 teaspoons onion powder

- 1 teaspoon fine sea salt

- Freshly ground black pepper

- 2 tablespoons finely chopped fresh parsley, optional

INSTRUCTIONS

Preheat the oven to 400 degrees Fahrenheit and line a large, rimmed baking sheet with parchment paper for easy clean-up.

Cut each potato in half lengthways, then in half lengthways again to make quarters, and then cut each half in half lengthways on the diagonal to make two wedges (you'll end up with 8 wedges per potato; make sure they are about the same thickness and size).

Place the sliced potatoes into a large bowl and cover them with hot water (I used hot water from the tap, but others have suggested that pipes can leach impurities into hot water, so it may be best to use cool tap water that has been heated on the stove). Let them soak for 10 minutes.

Drain the potatoes and lightly pat them dry with a lint-free tea towel. Place the potato wedges on the prepared pan and drizzle them with the olive oil. Sprinkle the garlic powder, onion powder, salt and a generous amount of pepper on top.

Toss until the potatoes are evenly coated in oil and spices, then arrange them in even columns across the pan so each wedge has a cut side against the pan. (If they don't all fit in an even layer across your pan, you'll need to use two pans for this recipe—divide them evenly across both pans, and rotate the pans when you flip the potatoes halfway through baking. They may be done baking earlier than specified below so keep an eye on them toward the end.)

Bake for 30 minutes, then flip the wedges over (use a spatula and you should be able to flip several at a time). Arrange them in an even layer and return the pan to the oven.

Bake until the wedges are deeply golden, crisp and easily pierced through by a fork, about 25 to 30 more minutes (the fries near the outside of my pan were done at 25, so I removed them and put the pan back in the oven for 5 more minutes to finish off the rest).

Sprinkle with parsley, if desired, and serve while hot.

Green Beans with Browned Butter Almondine

Ingredients

- 1 pound fresh green beans
- 3 tablespoons butter divided
- 1/2 cup slivered sliced almonds
- 1-2 tablespoons water or chicken broth
- 3/4 teaspoon kosher salt
- 1/2 teaspoon freshly ground black pepper
- Juice of 1 lemon to taste

Instructions

Trim the ends of the green beans and rinse well, set aside.

In a large skillet over medium low heat, melt 2 tablespoons of the butter. Add the almonds and cook for 2-3 minutes , stirring, until the nuts and butter become fragrantly nutty and begin to brown.

Add the green beans, and the kosher salt and freshly ground black pepper. Add 1 or 2 tablespoon of water or chicken broth to the pan to add more steam to the pan and cover with a lid and simmer until the beans are al denté, 4-5 minutes more, tossing the beans and almonds occasionally so the nuts don't burn.

Add the remaining tablespoon of butter with the juice of 1/2 off the lemon, and season with more salt and pepper and toss. Add more lemon juice to taste.

Panzanella for One

INGREDIENTS

- 2 tablespoons extra-virgin olive oil

- 2½ teaspoons balsamic vinegar

- 1 garlic clove, minced

- ½ teaspoon dried oregano

- Kosher salt

- 1 cucumber, peeled and chopped

- 1 cup cubed stale bread (from a rustic country loaf or baguette)

- 1 cup chopped tomato

- 4 ounces feta cheese, crumbled

- ¼ cup chopped red onion

- 6 Kalamata olives, pitted and chopped

DIRECTIONS

1. In a large bowl, combine the olive oil, vinegar, garlic, oregano and a pinch of salt. Whisk until emulsified. Add the cucumber, bread, tomato, feta, onion and olives. Use your hands to toss

the salad and evenly distribute the ingredients. Serve at room temperature.

Roasted Sweet Potatoes with Sriracha and Lime

INGREDIENTS

- Zest and juice of one lime

- ¼ cup coconut oil, melted

- 2 teaspoons kosher salt

- 2 teaspoons sriracha, plus more as needed

- 1½ pounds sweet potatoes, cut into 1-inch chunks

- Coarsely chopped fresh cilantro, for serving

DIRECTIONS

1. Preheat the oven to 425°F.

2. In a large bowl, whisk together the coconut oil, lime juice (save the zest for garnish), salt and sriracha.

3. Toss the sweet potatoes in the mixture. Roast in a single layer on two sheet pans until fork tender, 35 to 45 minutes, tossing occasionally and rotating the pans halfway through.

4. Transfer the roasted sweet potatoes to a serving platter. Top with the lime zest and a

handful of coarsely chopped fresh cilantro. Serve immediately.

Rainbow Vegetable Skewers

INGREDIENTS

- LEMON-PARSLEY DRESSING

- ⅓ cup freshly squeezed lemon juice

- Zest of 1 lemon

- 1 tablespoon Dijon mustard

- ½ cup extra-virgin olive oil

- ¼ cup chopped fresh parsley

- ¾ teaspoon garlic powder

- 1 pinch cayenne pepper

- Salt and freshly ground black pepper

- SKEWERS

- 3 red onions, cut into large pieces

- 2 summer squash, sliced

- 4 orange bell peppers, cut into squares

- 2 pints cherry tomatoes

- 2 zucchini, sliced

- 1 eggplant, cut into large cubes

- Salt and freshly ground black pepper

- 2 tablespoons chopped fresh parsley

DIRECTIONS

1. MAKE THE LEMON-PARSLEY DRESSING: In a medium bowl, whisk the lemon juice with the lemon zest and Dijon mustard to combine. Gradually add the olive oil, whisking well to combine. Add the parsley, garlic powder and cayenne; season with salt and pepper.

2. MAKE THE SKEWERS: Arrange the red onions tightly onto two skewers. Repeat with the other veggies.

3. Brush the skewers with the dressing on both sides and season with salt and pepper. Working in batches, cook on a preheated grill or grill pan until nicely charred, 3 to 5 minutes per side.

4. Garnish with parsley. Serve immediately with extra dressing on the side.

Melon Caprese Skewers

INGREDIENTS

- 1/2 cup Basil Vinaigrette

- 1 small cantaloupe scooped into balls

- 1 small honeydew scooped into balls

- 1 small seedless watermelon scooped into balls

- 20 fresh water-packed mozzarella balls drained

- 10 thin slices prosciutto cut in half lengthwise, gathered into ruffle

- Small wooden skewers about 4-6 inches long

- Maldon sea salt

- Freshly cracked black pepper

INSTRUCTIONS

Thread an assortment of the ingredients on the skewer - melon ball, basil leaf, mozzarella ball, ruffled prosciutto etc.

Arrange skewers on platter. Drizzle with basil vinaigrette and sprinkle with maldon sea salt and freshly cracked black pepper.

Creamy Sweet Corn Pappardelle

INGREDIENTS

- 2 tablespoons extra-virgin olive oil, divided

- ½ cup chopped yellow onion

- 5 ears corn, kernels cut from cobs (about 4 cups), divided

- 2 garlic cloves, crushed

- ½ cup raw cashews

- ¼ cup water, plus more if necessary

- 2 tablespoons fresh lemon juice

- ¼ teaspoon smoked paprika

- ½ teaspoon sea salt, plus more to taste

- Freshly ground black pepper

- 12 ounces pappardelle or pasta of choice

- 2 scallions, finely sliced

- 3 packed cups fresh spinach

- ½ cup sliced fresh basil, for serving (optional)

- Microgreens, for serving (optional)

DIRECTIONS

1. Heat 1 tablespoon of the olive oil in a medium skillet over medium heat. Add the onion and cook until soft, about 3 minutes. Add 1½ cups of the corn kernels and the whole crushed garlic cloves and cook until tender, about 3 minutes more. Transfer to a blender with the cashews, water, lemon juice, smoked paprika, ½ teaspoon sea salt and a few grinds of black pepper. Blend until creamy, adding more water as needed to create a pourable consistency. Set aside.

2. Bring a large pot of salted water to a boil. Prepare the pasta according to the instructions on the package, cooking until al dente. Reserve ½ cup of the hot pasta water, then drain.

3. Meanwhile, wipe out the skillet and heat the remaining 1 tablespoon olive oil over medium heat. Add the remaining 2½ cups corn, the scallions, a pinch of salt and a few grinds of black pepper; cook, stirring occasionally, until tender, about 3 minutes. Add the spinach, hot pasta, corn sauce and ¼ cup to ½ cup of the reserved pasta water, as needed, to create a creamy sauce. Season to taste and serve immediately with the sliced basil and microgreens, if using.

Burrata Salad with Stone Fruit and Asparagus

INGREDIENTS

- ¼ cup extra-virgin olive oil

- 2 tablespoons red-wine vinegar

- 1 tablespoon fresh lemon juice

- ¼ cup almonds, chopped and toasted

- 1 tablespoon chopped oregano

- ¼ teaspoon crushed red-pepper flakes

- Kosher salt and freshly ground black pepper

- 1 bunch asparagus

- 3 cups sugar snap peas

- 4 peaches, sliced

- 2 plums, sliced

- 3 cups cherries, halved and pitted

- ½ cup fresh mint leaves

- Two 8.8-ounce balls of burrata

DIRECTIONS

1. Bring a large pot of salted water to a boil. Have a bowl of ice water ready nearby.

2. Meanwhile, in a large bowl, whisk the olive oil with the red-wine vinegar and lemon juice. Stir in the almonds, oregano and red-pepper flakes; season with kosher salt and black pepper.

3. Working in batches, blanch the asparagus and sugar snap peas until bright green and slightly tender but still crunchy, about 30 seconds. Transfer each batch to the ice-water bath to cool, about 1 minute. Dry the vegetables on paper towels.

4. Add the asparagus, sugar snap peas, peaches, plums, cherries and mint leaves to the bowl of salad dressing and toss to coat.

5. Arrange the salad on a large serving platter and nestle in the burrata balls.

Gluten-Free Cauliflower Gnocchi Pomodoro

INGREDIENTS

- CAULIFLOWER GNOCCHI

- 1 head cauliflower, cut into florets (4 cups)

- 1 large russet potato, peeled and diced

- 3½ cups gluten-free all-purpose flour (such as Bob's Red Mill)

- ⅔ cup grated Parmesan cheese

- 1 teaspoon kosher salt

- ½ teaspoon freshly ground black pepper

- 2 large eggs, whisked lightly until combined

- Cornstarch

- POMODORO SAUCE

- 2 tablespoons extra-virgin olive oil

- 1 red onion, diced

- 3 garlic cloves, minced

- One 28-ounce can crushed tomatoes

- Kosher salt and freshly ground black pepper

- ½ teaspoon crushed red-pepper flakes

- 2 tablespoons unsalted butter

- ⅓ cup grated Parmesan cheese

- Basil, for serving

Spicy Whole Roasted Cauliflower

INGREDIENTS

- 1 tablespoon vegetable oil

- 1 head cauliflower

- 1½ cups plain Greek yogurt

- 1 lime, zested and juiced

- 2 tablespoons chile powder

- 1 tablespoon cumin

- 1 tablespoon garlic powder

- 1 teaspoon curry powder

- 2 teaspoons kosher salt

- 1 teaspoon black pepper

DIRECTIONS

1. Preheat the oven to 400° and lightly grease a small baking sheet with vegetable oil. Set aside.

2. Trim the base of the cauliflower to remove any green leaves and the woody stem.

3. In a medium bowl, combine the yogurt with the lime zest and juice, chile powder, cumin, garlic powder, curry powder, salt and pepper.

4. Dunk the cauliflower into the bowl and use a brush or your hands to smear the marinade evenly over its surface. (Excess marinade can be stored in the refrigerator in an airtight container for up to three days and used with meat, fish or other veggies.)

5. Place the cauliflower on the prepared baking sheet and roast until the surface is dry and

lightly browned, 30 to 40 minutes. The marinade will make a crust on the surface of the cauliflower.

6. Let the cauliflower cool for 10 minutes before cutting it into wedges and serving alongside a big green salad.

Chocolate Chip Cookie in a Mug

INGREDIENTS

- 2 tablespoons butter

- 2 tablespoons sugar

- 1 tablespoon light brown sugar

- 1 egg

- ¼ teaspoon pure vanilla extract

- ⅓ cup all-purpose flour

- ¼ teaspoon baking powder

- Pinch of salt

- 2 tablespoons chocolate chips

DIRECTIONS

1. To begin, in a large mug, melt the butter in the microwave, about 15 to 30 seconds. Add in the sugar as well as the light brown sugar and stir to combine. Next, add the egg and vanilla extract, and then whisk together.

2. Next, add the flour, baking powder and salt to the mug; stir to combine. Continue by stirring in the chocolate chips.

3. Finally, put the mug in the microwave and heat for about 1 to 2 minutes until cooked. Another way to check is to insert a toothpick into the center and make sure it comes out clean. Once cooked throughout, serve immediately and enjoy.

Cacio e Pepe

INGREDIENTS

- 12 ounces spaghetti

- 4 tablespoons unsalted butter, at room temperature

- 1 tablespoon extra-virgin olive oil

- ⅔ cup grated Pecorino Romano cheese

- Kosher salt and freshly ground black pepper, to taste

DIRECTIONS

1. Bring a large pot of salted water to a boil. Add the spaghetti and cook until just al dente, 8 to 10 minutes.

2. While the pasta cooks, mash the soft butter with the olive oil and Pecorino in a large bowl to form a paste.

3. When the pasta is cooked, reserve ½ cup of the pasta cooking water and drain the spaghetti. Add the spaghetti directly to the bowl with the butter mixture. Toss well to coat, adding the pasta water as needed to make a thick, creamy sauce that coats the pasta strands. Season to taste with salt and lots of freshly ground black pepper. Divide the pasta among four plates; serve immediately.

Pasta Limone

INGREDIENTS

- 12 ounces spaghetti, linguine or bucatini

- 2 leeks, thinly sliced

- 2 garlic cloves, thinly sliced

- Zest and juice of 1 lemon, plus more lemon zest for serving

- 3 sprigs basil, plus more for serving

- 1 teaspoon kosher salt

- ¾ teaspoon freshly ground black pepper, plus more for serving

- 1 cup grated Parmesan cheese

DIRECTIONS

1. Combine the pasta, 4½ cups water, leeks, garlic, lemon zest, basil, salt and pepper in a large skillet with 2-inch sides.

2. Bring the water to a boil and cook, stirring occasionally, until the water is nearly gone and the pasta is fully cooked, 8 to 10 minutes.

3. Add the lemon juice and Parmesan, and toss to combine. Season with salt and pepper to taste. Garnish with basil leaves and lemon zest.

Spicy Roasted Brussels Sprouts

INGREDIENTS

- 1½ pounds brussels sprouts

- ½ cup extra-virgin olive oil

- ¼ cup rice-wine vinegar

- ¼ cup honey

- 2 tablespoons Sriracha, or more to taste

- Kosher salt and freshly ground black pepper

DIRECTIONS

1. Preheat the oven to 400°F. Trim the base away from the brussels sprouts and discard. Cut the sprouts in half.

2. In a large bowl, whisk the olive oil with the vinegar, honey and Sriracha to combine. Add the brussels sprouts and toss until they are fully coated. Season with salt and pepper to taste.

3. Spread the brussels sprouts on a baking sheet, cut sides down. Pour any extra olive-oil mixture

onto the pan and tilt the pan around to distribute it.

4. Roast until the sprouts are crispy on the outside and golden and caramelized on the cut sides, 20 to 30 minutes. Serve immediately.

Baked Mac-and-Cheese Bites

INGREDIENTS

- 1 pound small elbow pasta

- 3 tablespoons unsalted butter

- 1 small onion, minced

- 2 garlic cloves, minced

- ¼ cup all-purpose flour

- 2½ cups whole milk

- ¼ teaspoon cayenne pepper (optional)

- Salt and freshly ground black pepper

- 2 cups grated white cheddar cheese

- 2 cups grated yellow cheddar cheese, divided

DIRECTIONS

1. Preheat the oven to 375°F. Grease two mini-muffin pans with nonstick cooking spray.

2. Bring a large pot of salted water to a boil. Add the elbow pasta and cook according to the package instructions, about 7 to 9 minutes. Drain.

3. In a large pot, melt the butter over medium heat. Add the onion and sauté until translucent, 4 to 5 minutes. Add the garlic and cook until fragrant, 1 minute more.

4. Sprinkle the flour into the pot and stir to combine. Cook for 2 minutes, stirring constantly.

5. Add the milk and whisk well to combine. Bring the mixture to a simmer over medium-low heat, stirring occasionally.

6. Season the sauce with the cayenne pepper (if using), salt and pepper. Remove the pot from

the heat and stir in the white cheddar and 1½ cups of the yellow cheddar. Stir until the mixture is melted.

7. Stir in the cooked pasta and mix until it is evenly coated with the sauce. Scoop 1½ to 2 tablespoons of the mac-and-cheese mixture into each cavity of the prepared pans.

8. Sprinkle a few pieces of yellow cheddar on top of each mac-and-cheese bite and then transfer the pans to the oven. Bake until the cheese is melted and the bites become golden, 17 to 20 minutes.

9. Let the bites cool for 15 minutes before unmolding and serving. Serve hot or at room temperature. Store leftovers in an airtight container in the refrigerator for up to two days.

Cheater's White Wine Coq au Vin

INGREDIENTS

- 3 pounds chicken (8 pieces total—thighs, breasts and drumsticks)

- Kosher salt and freshly ground black pepper

- 2 tablespoons unsalted butter

- 4 strips bacon, diced

- 1 large sweet onion, diced

- 3 garlic cloves, minced

- 1 pint cremini mushrooms, sliced

- 2 cups dry white wine

- 1 tablespoon whole-grain mustard

- ½ cup heavy cream

- ¼ cup chopped fresh parsley

DIRECTIONS

1. Season the chicken with salt and pepper. In a large skillet, melt the butter over medium heat. Add the chicken to the skillet and cook until it's well browned, about 4 minutes per side.

2. Remove the chicken from the skillet and set aside. Add the bacon to the skillet and cook until the fat begins to render, about 3 minutes.

3. Add the onion and sauté until it becomes translucent, about 5 minutes. Add the garlic and mushrooms, and sauté until the mushrooms are tender, 5 to 6 minutes.

4. Add the browned chicken back to the skillet. Pour the wine into the skillet, stir in the mustard and bring the mixture to a simmer over medium-low heat.

5. Cover the skillet and simmer until the chicken is almost fully cooked, 15 to 20 minutes.

6. Uncover the skillet and add the cream. Simmer until the sauce thickens and the chicken is fully cooked, 8 to 10 minutes.

7. Garnish with parsley and serve immediately.

Cheese and Bacon Baked Potatoes

INGREDIENTS

- 4 large russet potatoes

- 4 tablespoons butter, softened

- Salt and freshly ground black pepper

- ½ cup shredded cheddar cheese

- ½ cup chopped cooked bacon, crumbled

DIRECTIONS

1. Preheat the oven to 400°F. Line a baking sheet with aluminum foil.

2. Use a sharp knife to cut the entire top of the potato into thin crosswise slices (about ⅛-inch thick), stopping about three-quarters of the way down the potato so the base stays in tact and the pieces remain attached to the base.

3. Rub 1 tablespoon butter evenly across the top of each potato. Season the potatoes with salt and pepper, and then place them on the prepared baking sheet.

4. Roast the potatoes until they are golden and easily pierced with a fork, 20 to 25 minutes.

5. Remove the baking sheet from the oven and sprinkle each baked potato with 2 tablespoons shredded cheese and 2 tablespoons bacon. Push some of the toppings between the potato slices. Return the baking sheet to the oven and cook until the bacon is crisp and the cheese is melted, 5 to 7 minutes more.

6. Let the potatoes cool for 5 minutes before serving.

Slow-Cooker Chicken Teriyaki

- INGREDIENTS

- 4 boneless, skinless chicken breasts

- 1 onion

- 3 cloves garlic

- 1 tablespoon fresh ginger

- ½ cup soy sauce

- ⅓ cup honey

- ⅓ cup rice vinegar

- ¼ cup scallions, sliced

- 3 tablespoons sesame seeds

- 2 cups white rice, steamed (for serving)

DIRECTIONS

1. Place the chicken breasts into your slow cooker.

2. Top the chicken with the onion, garlic and ginger.

3. Add the soy sauce, honey and rice vinegar to the slow cooker; season with salt and pepper.

4. Cook on low for 6 hours. Shred the chicken with two forks.

5. Garnish the cooked chicken with sliced scallions and sesame seeds. Serve with the steamed rice.

Balsamic Cranberry Roast Chicken

INGREDIENTS

- 2 cloves garlic

- ¼ cup balsamic vinegar

- 3 tablespoons extra-virgin olive oil

- 1 tablespoon soy sauce

- 1½ cups cranberries, divided

- 8 pieces chicken (thighs, drumsticks or a mixture)

- Nonstick spray, as needed

- Kosher salt and freshly ground black pepper

- 1 tablespoon chopped fresh thyme, plus extra sprigs for finishing

- 1 tablespoon chopped fresh rosemary, plus extra sprigs for finishing

DIRECTIONS

1. In the bowl of a food processor or blender, process the garlic, balsamic vinegar, olive oil, soy sauce and ½ cup of the cranberries until smooth.

2. Place the chicken pieces in a large zip-top plastic bag and pour the marinade over the

chicken. Close the bag and refrigerate for 30 minutes to 1 hour.

3. Preheat the oven to 375°F. Lightly grease a large oven-safe skillet or casserole dish with nonstick spray.

4. Remove the chicken from the bag, reserving the marinade. Place the chicken pieces in the skillet or dish, skin side down, and season with salt, pepper, thyme and rosemary. Sprinkle the remaining 1 cup cranberries around the pan.

5. Roast the chicken until the skin begins to brown and the meat is nearly cooked through, 20 to 25 minutes. Flip the chicken and brush each piece generously with the reserved marinade. Discard the remaining marinade.

6. Raise the oven temperature to 425°F and cook until the chicken skin is crispy, 5 to 8 more minutes. Serve immediately.

Cauliflower Fried Rice

INGREDIENTS

- FRIED RICE

- 1 head cauliflower, cut into florets

- 2 tablespoons neutral oil (such as vegetable, coconut or peanut)

- 1 bunch scallions, thinly sliced

- 3 garlic cloves, minced

- 1 tablespoon minced fresh ginger

- 2 carrots, peeled and diced

- 2 celery stalks, diced

- 1 red bell pepper, diced

- 1 cup frozen peas

- 2 tablespoons rice vinegar

- 3 tablespoons soy sauce

- 2 teaspoons Sriracha, or more to taste

- GARNISHES

- 1 tablespoon neutral oil (such as vegetable, coconut or peanut)

- 4 eggs

- Salt and freshly ground black pepper

- 4 tablespoons chopped fresh cilantro

- 4 tablespoons thinly sliced scallions

- 4 teaspoons sesame seeds

DIRECTIONS

1. MAKE THE FRIED RICE: In the bowl of a food processor, pulse the cauliflower until the mixture resembles rice, 2 to 3 minutes. Set aside.

2. In a large skillet, heat the oil over medium heat. Add the scallions, garlic and ginger, and stir-fry until fragrant, about 1 minute.

3. Add the carrots, celery and red bell pepper, and stir-fry until the vegetables are tender, 9 to 11 minutes.

4. Add the cauliflower rice and stir-fry until it begins to turn golden, 3 to 5 minutes more. Stir in the frozen peas and toss well to combine.

5. Add the rice vinegar, soy sauce and Sriracha, and toss to combine. Set aside.

6. MAKE THE GARNISHES: In a medium skillet, heat the oil over medium-high heat. Crack the eggs directly into the pan and cook until the whites are set but the yolks are still runny, 3 to 4 minutes. Season each with salt and pepper.

7. To serve, divide the cauliflower rice among four plates and top each with a fried egg. Garnish each plate with 1 tablespoon cilantro, 1 tablespoon scallions and 1 teaspoon sesame seeds. Serve immediately.

General Tso's Cauliflower

INGREDIENTS

- CAULIFLOWER

- ½ cup all-purpose flour

- ⅓ cup cornstarch

- ¾ teaspoon baking powder

- 1 teaspoon salt

- 2 eggs

- 3 tablespoons soy sauce

- 1 tablespoon rice vinegar

- ½ cup neutral oil (like peanut or vegetable)

- 1 head cauliflower, cut into bite-size florets

- SAUCE

- 2 teaspoons sesame oil

- 6 scallions, white parts finely chopped, green parts chopped into 1-inch pieces and reserved

- 3 cloves garlic, minced

- 1 tablespoon minced ginger

- 5 small dried chiles (optional)

- ¼ cup vegetable broth

- ¼ cup soy sauce

- 3 tablespoons rice vinegar

- 2 tablespoons mirin

- 3 tablespoons sugar

- 1 tablespoon cornstarch

- Sesame seeds, for garnish (optional)

- Steamed rice, for serving

DIRECTIONS

1. PREPARE THE CAULIFLOWER: In a medium bowl, whisk the flour, cornstarch, baking powder and salt to combine. In a liquid measuring cup,

whisk the eggs, soy sauce and vinegar to combine. Slowly pour the egg mixture into the flour, whisking constantly. You should end up with a thick but still dip-able batter (thin with a little water if it's too thick).

2. Heat the oil in a medium cast iron skillet over medium-high heat until very hot (you can test it by dropping a small amount of batter into the oil—it should immediately sizzle and float).

3. Dip each piece of cauliflower in the batter to fully coat, then carefully place in the oil. Pan-fry the cauliflower until golden on all sides, about 5 minutes. Transfer to a plate lined with paper towels to drain the excess oil.

4. MAKE THE SAUCE: Meanwhile, in a medium saucepan, heat the sesame oil over medium heat. Add the finely-chopped scallion whites, garlic,

ginger and chiles (if using), and cook until fragrant, about 2 minutes.

5. Add the broth, soy sauce, rice vinegar and mirin, and bring to a simmer over medium heat. Simmer for about 5 minutes.

6. In a small bowl, whisk the sugar and cornstarch to combine. Pour about ¼ cup of the hot sauce over the cornstarch mixture, whisking constantly until the mixture is smooth and lump free. Return the mixture to the pot and bring to a simmer. Stir in the large pieces of green scallion.

7. Cook, stirring occasionally, until the mixture thickens, 7 to 9 minutes more.

8. Add the cauliflower to the pot and toss to coat until the cauliflower is rewarmed, about 5 minutes. Serve immediately, garnished with sesame seeds and served with a side of steamed rice.

Easy One-Pan Ratatouille

INGREDIENTS

- 5 tablespoons olive oil

- 2 garlic cloves, smashed

- 2 sprigs oregano

- 1 cup tomato puree (or tomato sauce)

- 1 small eggplant, thickly sliced

- 1 medium red onion, thickly sliced

- 2 medium summer squash, thickly sliced

- 2 medium zucchini, thickly sliced

- 2 small red bell peppers, sides cut off and halved

- 3 medium tomatoes, thickly sliced

- 2 tablespoons thyme leaves

- Salt and freshly ground black pepper

DIRECTIONS

1. Preheat the oven to 375°F. Place four individual baking dishes or one 9-inch square baking dish on a baking sheet.

2. In a small pot, heat the olive oil and garlic over medium-low heat. Cook until fragrant, about 1 minute. Remove the pot from the heat, add the oregano and let steep for 15 minutes. Remove and discard the garlic and oregano.

3. Drizzle 2 teaspoons of the olive oil into the base of each small baking dish (or 2 tablespoons into the base of the larger baking dish).

4. Spread 2 tablespoons tomato puree on the base of each baking dish (or ¼ cup on the base of the larger baking dish).

5. Layer the eggplant, onion, summer squash, zucchini, pepper and tomato in the prepared baking dishes. Stagger the slices slightly and don't worry about being perfect or matchy--just make sure they are packed in tightly.

6. Brush the remaining tomato puree on top, then drizzle evenly with the remaining oil. Sprinkle with thyme and season with salt and pepper.

7. Roast until tender and beginning to brown at the surface and edges, 25 to 30 minutes. Cool for 5 to 10 minutes before serving.

Ina Garten's Updated Chicken Marbella

INGREDIENTS

- ½ cup good olive oil

- ½ cup good red wine vinegar

- 1½ cups large pitted prunes, such as Sunsweet

- 1 cup large green olives, pitted, such as Cerignola

- ½ cup capers, including the juices (3½ ounces)

- 6 bay leaves

- 1½ heads of garlic—cloves separated, peeled and minced

- ¼ cup dried oregano

- Kosher salt and freshly ground black pepper

- Two 4-pound chickens, backs removed and cut in 8 pieces

- ½ cup light brown sugar, lightly packed

- 1 cup dry white wine, such as Pinot Grigio

DIRECTIONS

1. Combine the olive oil, vinegar, prunes, olives, capers, bay leaves, garlic, oregano, 2 tablespoons salt and 2 teaspoons pepper in a large bowl. Add the chicken to the marinade. (You can also place the chicken and marinade in a 2-gallon plastic storage bag and squeeze out the air to make sure the chicken is fully covered with the marinade.) Refrigerate overnight, turning occasionally to be sure the marinade is getting into all the chicken pieces.

2. Preheat the oven to 350°F. Place the chicken, skin side up, along with the marinade in one layer in a large (15-by-18-inch) roasting pan, sprinkle with the brown sugar, 2 teaspoons salt and 1 teaspoon pepper and pour the wine around (not over!) the chicken. Roast until the internal temperature of the chicken is 145°F, 45 to 55 minutes.

3. Remove the pan from the oven, cover tightly with aluminum foil and allow to rest for 10 to 15 minutes. Discard the bay leaves. Transfer the chicken, prunes and olives to a serving platter, sprinkle with salt and serve hot with the pan juices.

Skillet Gnocchi with Sausage and Broccoli Rabe

INGREDIENTS

- 1 pound store-bought gnocchi

- 2 tablespoons unsalted butter

- 1 sweet onion, sliced

- 2 garlic cloves, minced

- 1 pound cooked Italian sausage, sliced

- 1 bunch broccoli rabe, cut into bite-size pieces

- ½ cup chicken broth

- Salt and freshly ground black pepper

- ½ teaspoon red-pepper flakes (optional)

- ½ cup grated Parmesan cheese

- ¼ cup chopped fresh parsley

DIRECTIONS

1. Bring a large pot of salted water to a boil. Add the gnocchi and cook until the pasta floats to the surface, 4 to 5 minutes. Drain the gnocchi.

2. In a large skillet, melt the butter over medium heat. Add the onion and sauté until translucent, 4 to 5 minutes. Add the garlic and sauté until fragrant, 1 minute more.

3. Add the sausage and cook until it begins to brown, 3 to 4 minutes. Add the broccoli rabe and chicken broth, and bring to a simmer.

4. Continue to cook, tossing frequently, until the broccoli rabe is wilted and tender, about 5 minutes. Season with salt, pepper and red-pepper flakes (if desired).

5. Stir in the gnocchi, Parmesan and parsley, and toss well until combined. Serve immediately.

Spaghetti with Avocado Pasta Sauce

INGREDIENTS

- 12 ounces spaghetti

- 2 avocados--halved, pitted and peeled

- 1 garlic clove, smashed

- 1 bunch scallions, roughly chopped

- Juice of 1 lemon

- ¼ cup extra-virgin olive oil

- Salt and freshly ground black pepper

- ½ cup chopped parsley, for garnish

DIRECTIONS

1. Bring a large pot of salted water to a boil. Add the spaghetti and cook until al dente, 6 to 8 minutes.

2. While the pasta cooks, make the sauce: In the bowl of a food processor, pulse the avocados, garlic, scallions, lemon juice and olive oil until smooth.

3. When the pasta is tender, reserve ½ cup of the cooking water, then drain the pasta. Add the

reserved water to the avocado mixture and process until smooth.

4. Add the sauce to the pasta and toss to coat. Season with salt and pepper. To serve, portion the pasta onto plates and garnish with parsley.

Cinnamon-Roll Pie Crust

INGREDIENTS

- 1 package pie crust

- 4 tablespoons butter, melted

- ½ cup brown sugar

- 2 teaspoons cinnamon

- ½ teaspoon pure vanilla extract

DIRECTIONS

1. On a lightly floured surface, roll out the pie crust a few times to even it out to about ½-inch thickness.

2. In a small bowl, mix the butter with the sugar, cinnamon and vanilla extract to combine. Spoon the mixture into the center of the crust. Use a spatula to spread it evenly over the entire crust.

3. Starting with the side closest to you, roll the crust into a tight spiral. Cut the finished spiral into ½-inch-thick pieces.

4. On a lightly floured surface, use a rolling pin to roll each piece into a ¼-inch-thick round. Place the pieces in a pie plate, overlapping them

slightly and pressing to seal. (If the pieces aren't sticking together well, use a little water to help "glue" them.)

5. Continue placing rounds of dough in the pie plate until the entire plate is full; trim any excess hanging over the edge. Use the tines of a fork to press indentations all around the edge. Chill the crust well before filling and baking, and bake according to your preferred pie recipe.

The Best Potatoes au Gratin Ever

INGREDIENTS

- 5 tablespoons unsalted butter, divided

- 1 sweet onion, thinly sliced

- 3 garlic cloves, minced

- 1 tablespoon grainy mustard

- 2 cups half-and-half

- 2 pounds potatoes, peeled and thinly sliced

- Salt and freshly ground black pepper

- ½ teaspoon freshly grated nutmeg

- ¾ cup grated Gruyère cheese

DIRECTIONS

1. Preheat the oven to 375°F. Grease a 9-by-13-inch casserole dish with 1 tablespoon of the butter.

2. In a large pot, heat the remaining 4 tablespoons of butter over medium heat. Add in the onion and sauté until tender and translucent, about 4 to 5 minutes. Add the garlic and cook until fragrant, 1 minute more.

3. Stir in the mustard. Then add the half-and-half and bring to a simmer. Add the potatoes and simmer for 4 to 5 minutes. Season with the salt, pepper and nutmeg.

4. Pour the potato mixture into the prepared casserole dish and spread into an even layer. Top with the cheese in an even layer. (The dish can be stored, covered, in the refrigerator at this point if you want to prepare it ahead.)

5. Bake until the cheese is golden, the sauce is bubbly and the potatoes are easily pierced with a

fork, 25 to 30 minutes (add 5 to 7 minutes if baking after storing in the refrigerator). Let cool 5 minutes before serving warm. Prepare thy tastebuds.

Mini Mason Jar Apple Pies

INGREDIENTS

- FILLING

- 4 tablespoons unsalted butter

- 2 Honeycrisp apples, peeled and chopped (or other baking apple, such as Granny Smith or McIntosh)

- ½ cup brown sugar

- 3 tablespoons all-purpose flour

- 2 teaspoons cinnamon

- ½ teaspoon ginger

- ½ teaspoon cloves

- 1 teaspoon pure vanilla extract

- ASSEMBLY

- 2 packages store-bought pie dough (4 circles total)

- 1 egg

- 1 tablespoon water

- 1½ teaspoons turbinado sugar

DIRECTIONS

1. MAKE THE FILLING: Preheat the oven to 400°F. Have ready six ¼ pint (½ cup) mason jars on a baking sheet.

2. In a large skillet, melt the butter over medium heat. Add the apples and sauté until nearly tender, about 5 minutes. Add the sugar, flour, cinnamon, ginger, cloves and vanilla extract, and sauté for about 2 minutes more. Let the mixture cool to room temperature.

3. ASSEMBLE THE PIES: On a lightly floured surface, roll out the pie dough until it is flat and slightly thinner than it originally was. Cut the dough into six 3-inch circles and six 2-inch circles.

4. Press a 3-inch circle into a mason jar, pressing it firmly to the base and sides and taking care not to poke holes in the dough. Trim any excess from the top edge with a paring knife. Repeat with the remaining 3-inch circles and jars.

5. Scoop the cooled filling into the pastry-lined jars, mounding it about ½ an inch over the top rim. Place the 2-inch rounds over the filling and tuck the edges under so they meet the edge of the jar. Crimp the edges with your fingers or a fork. Chill the pies for 10 minutes.

6. While the pies chill, whisk the egg and water together to combine. Use a pastry brush to brush the egg wash over each pie top, then sprinkle the top of each with ½ teaspoon turbinado sugar. Cut small vents into the top of each pie with a paring knife.

7. Bake until the pies are golden brown, 20 to 25 minutes. Cool for at least 10 minutes before serving.

Baby Blooming Onion Recipe

INGREDIENTS

- DIPPING SAUCE

- ½ cup sour cream

- ¼ cup mayonnaise

- 1 tablespoon prepared horseradish

- ½ teaspoon garlic powder

- 1 teaspoon smoked paprika

- Salt and freshly ground black pepper, to taste

- ONIONS

- 2 pounds cipollini onions, peeled

- 1½ cups buttermilk

- 2 cups all-purpose flour

- 2 teaspoons salt

- 1 teaspoon black pepper

- 1 teaspoon garlic powder

- ½ teaspoon cayenne pepper

- ¾ teaspoon baking powder

- Vegetable oil, as needed for frying

DIRECTIONS

1. MAKE THE DIPPING SAUCE: In a medium bowl, whisk the sour cream with the mayonnaise, horseradish, garlic powder, paprika, salt and pepper to combine. Set aside.

2. MAKE THE ONIONS: Slice an onion in half vertically, but don't cut all the way through to the base. The idea is to keep the bottom intact. Turn the onion 45 degrees, slice vertically again and repeat until you end up with what looks like little rectangles of onion, still attached at the base. Repeat with the remaining onions.

3. Loosen the onions a little by wiggling them around to separate the pieces slightly and create space between them. Place the buttermilk in a shallow dish and then add the onions to it. Toss well and massage the onions to get the buttermilk into the score marks.

4. In a medium-size shallow dish, whisk the flour with the salt, pepper, garlic powder, cayenne and baking powder to combine.

5. Heat 3 inches of oil in a wide pot over medium-high heat until it reads 350°F on a thermometer.

6. Working one at a time, remove an onion from the buttermilk and dredge fully in the flour mixture, working again to make sure the breading gets into the score marks.

7. Working in batches, fry the onions until they're golden and crisp, flipping them over halfway through cooking, about 8 to 10 minutes. Set the cooked onions on paper towels to absorb the excess oil.

8. Serve immediately with the dipping sauce.

Paella in the oven

Ingredients

- 400g can chopped tomatoes

- 600ml chicken stock

- 1 tsp smoked paprika

- good pinch of saffron

- 1 onion , chopped

- 1 garlic clove , crushed or finely chopped

- 2 tbsp olive oil

- 300g paella rice

- 4 chicken thighs (skin on or boneless), cut in half

- 200g chorizo , sliced

- 150g raw king prawns , leave the shell on a few if you prefer

- good handful of frozen peas

- 1 lemon , quartered (optional)

Method

STEP 1

Heat oven to 220C/200C fan/gas 8. Put the chopped tomatoes (including their juice), stock, paprika and saffron in a large heatproof jug or bowl and microwave for about 5 mins on high until steaming hot.

STEP 2

Tip the onion and garlic into a generous roasting tin or ovenproof dish, drizzle over the oil and mix to coat. Cook in the oven for 20 mins until beginning to brown.

STEP 3

Stir in the rice, chicken, chorizo and hot stock mixture, season well and return to the oven for 20 mins (don't cover).

STEP 4

Stir in the peeled prawns and peas, dot any shell-on prawns on top, and return to the oven for 5-10 mins until the rice, chicken and prawns are cooked through. If serving with lemon, a nice touch is to pop the lemon slices on top of the paella for the last 5 mins of cooking, to make them hot and juicy. Check the seasoning and serve at once.

Umami gravy

Ingredients

- 100g unsalted butter

- 20g salted anchovies , chopped

- 400ml beef stock (the best quality you can get)

- 20ml sherry vinegar

Method

STEP 1

Melt the butter in a pan over a high heat. Bubble, swirling the pan until it turns a nut brown colour. Add the anchovies, and sizzle for 1-2 mins until they dissolve.

STEP 2

Add the stock and vinegar. Bring to the boil and reduce for around 20 mins to the desired consistency. Sieve and serve.

Soft burger buns

Ingredients

- 200ml whole milk , plus extra for brushing

- 50g unsalted butter

- 500g plain flour , plus extra for dusting

- 1 tbsp caster sugar

- 7g sachet fast-action dried yeast

- 1 egg , beaten

- sesame seeds (optional)

Method

STEP 1

Put the milk, butter and 100ml water in a pan and gently heat until the butter is melted. Set aside to cool until just warm.

STEP 2

Tip the flour, sugar, yeast and 1 tsp salt into a large bowl and gradually work in the milk mixture, then the egg, until you have a smooth dough. Tip the dough onto a floured surface or into a stand mixer fitted with a dough hook and knead until elastic and shiny. Divide into 12 (about 80g each) pieces and roll into tight balls. Transfer to baking trays lined with baking parchment, leaving plenty of space between them, and put in a warm place to prove for 30-45 mins.

STEP 3

Heat oven to 200C/180C fan/gas 6. Press the rolls down gently using your hands, then brush over some milk and scatter over the sesame seeds, if you like (or, dust with some flour). Bake for 10-12 mins until risen and lightly golden. Leave to cool completely, then serve. Make up to two days ahead and keep in an airtight container.

Dalgona coffee

Ingredients

- 3 tbsp instant coffee

- 2 tbsp sugar

- 400-500ml milk (we used whole milk)

Method

STEP 1

Whisk the coffee, sugar and 3 tbsp boiling water in a bowl for approximately 5 mins until the mixture is thick and fluffy with stiff peaks. This is easiest done using an electric whisk but can be done by hand.

STEP 2

For hot coffee, heat the milk and pour into two heatproof glasses. For cold coffee, pour the cold milk into two glasses. Divide the coffee mixture in half and spoon evenly on top of the glasses. Serve and stir thoroughly before drinking.

Pizza with homemade sauce

Ingredients

- 300g strong white bread flour , plus extra for dusting

- 1 tsp instant yeast

- 1 tbsp olive oil

- For the tomato sauce

- 1 tbsp olive oil , plus a drizzle

- 2 garlic cloves , crushed

- 200ml passata

- For the topping

- 8 mozzarella pearls , halved

- small bunch fresh basil

Method

STEP 1

Tip the flour into a bowl, then stir in the yeast and 1 tsp salt. Make a well in the centre and pour in 200ml warm water (make sure it's not too hot) along with the oil. Stir together with a wooden spoon until you have a soft, fairly wet dough.

STEP 2

Tip the dough out onto a lightly floured surface and knead for 5 mins until smooth. Cover with a tea towel and set aside for an hour or so or until the dough has puffed up and doubled in size. You can also leave the rough, unkneaded dough in the bowl, cover with a tea towel and leave in the fridge overnight and the dough will continue to prove on its own.

STEP 3

Meanwhile, make the tomato sauce. Put the oil in a small pan and fry the garlic briefly (don't let it brown), then add the passata and simmer everything until the sauce thickens a little. Leave to cool.

STEP 4

Once the dough has risen, knead it quickly in the bowl to knock it back, then tip out onto a lightly floured surface and cut into two balls. Roll out each ball into a large teardrop that is very thin and about 25cm across (teardrop shapes fit baking sheets more easily than rounds).

STEP 5

Heat oven to 240C/220C fan/ gas 9 with a large baking sheet inside. Lift one of the bases onto another floured baking sheet. Smooth the sauce over the base with the back of a spoon, scatter over half the mozzarella, drizzle with olive oil and season. Put the pizza, still on its baking sheet, on top of the hot sheet in the oven and bake for 8-10 mins until crisp.

Pollo en pepitoria

Ingredients

- good pinch of saffron

- 4 tbsp extra virgin olive oil

- 6 garlic cloves

- 35g blanched almonds

- 30g stale bread , torn

- 2 tbsp parsley , chopped, plus extra to serve

- 8 skin-on and bone-in chicken thighs

- 1 onion , finely chopped

- 1 carrot , chopped

- 1 celery stick, chopped

- 250ml dry sherry

- 350ml chicken stock

- 1 cinnamon stick , broken in two

- pinch of ground cloves

- 2 bay leaves

- 2 eggs , hard-boiled, shelled and halved

- 2 tbsp flaked almonds , toasted

Method

STEP 1

Put the saffron in a small bowl with 75ml of just-boiled water. Stir and set aside. Heat 2 tbsp of the oil in a broad, shallow casserole dish. Cook the garlic until pale gold in colour, then add the blanched almonds and bread, and continue to fry until everything is golden. Tip into a food processor with some salt and pepper and the parsley, and whizz together.

STEP 2

Heat 2 more tbsp of the oil in the pan and brown the chicken all over, seasoning as you cook. Put in a bowl and set aside.

STEP 3

Remove all but about 2 tbsp of chicken fat from the pan and cook the onion, carrot and celery until golden. Add the sherry, stirring to dislodge any brown bits that have stuck to the pan. Pour in the stock and the saffron (with its water), and bring to the boil, then turn the heat down to a simmer. Add the spices and bay leaves, and put the chicken back in the pan with any juices. Season and gently cook the chicken for about 40 mins with the lid on.

STEP 4

Transfer the chicken to a bowl again, leaving the sauce in the pan, and cover with foil to keep warm. Remove the yolks from the eggs and roughly chop the whites. Mash the egg yolks in a small bowl and gradually mix in a couple of tbsp of the sauce. Bring the remaining sauce to the boil to reduce a bit (you want it to just coat the chicken), then turn the heat down. Remove the bay and cinnamon stick. Add the egg yolks and cook for a few mins until the mixture has thickened. Stir in the almond mixture that you made earlier (this will thicken the sauce, too). Put the chicken back in the pan and heat it for about 3 mins, spooning the sauce over it. Season to taste.

STEP 5

Scatter over the extra parsley, the almonds pieces and the chopped egg whites (if you're going to use them). You can serve this straight from the dish with some rice, if you like.

Ravioli lasagne

Ingredients

- oil , for frying

- 6 sausages (we used Italian sausages with herbs and fennel)

- 2 x 400g cans chopped tomatoes with garlic & basil

- 200g baby spinach

- 500g spinach & ricotta ravioli (or any flavour you like)

- 75g mixture of grated cheddar and mozzarella

Method

STEP 1

Heat a drizzle of oil in a pan. Squeeze the sausagemeat from the skins and fry until browned, using a wooden spoon to break it up.

Add the tomatoes and half a can of water and season. Simmer for 20 mins.

STEP 2

Meanwhile, put the spinach in a colander. Pour over boiled water from the kettle to wilt. Leave to cool, then squeeze out as much of the excess water as you can.

STEP 3

Heat the oven to 200C/180C fan/gas 6. Spoon a third of the sauce into a medium baking dish (about 18 x 20cm). Top with a third of the spinach and a third of the ravioli, then scatter over some of the cheese. Repeat the layers twice, making sure the final layer of ravioli is nestled into the sauce. Bake for 35-40 mins until bubbling and hot all the way through. Cover if the top starts to get too dark. Will keep in the freezer for up to two months.

Slow cooker gammon in cola

Ingredients

- 1.5-1.8kg unsmoked boneless gammon joint

- 2l cola (not diet)

- 1 carrot, peeled and chopped

- 1 onion, peeled and quartered

- 1 stick celery, chopped

- 1 cinnamon stick

- ½ tbsp peppercorns

- 1 bay leaf

- For the glaze

- 150ml maple syrup

- 2 tbsp wholegrain mustard

- 2 tbsp red wine vinegar

- pinch of ground cloves or five-spice

Method

STEP 1

Set your slow cooker to medium. Place the gammon joint in and cover with the cola. Add 1 chopped carrot, 1 quartered onion, 1 chopped celery stick, 1 cinnamon stick, ½ tbsp peppercorns and 1 bay leaf.

STEP 2

Cook for 5½ hrs on low until the gammon is tender but still holding its shape, topping up with boiling water if necessary to keep the gammon fully covered.

STEP 3

Carefully pour the liquid away, then let the ham cool a little while you heat the oven to 190C/170C fan/gas 5. Lift the ham into a roasting tin, then cut away the skin leaving behind an even layer of fat. Score the fat all over in a criss-cross pattern.

STEP 4

Mix the maple syrup, mustard, vinegar and ground cloves or five-spice in a jug. Pour half over the fat, roast for 15 mins, then pour over the rest and return to the oven for another 30 mins.

STEP 5

Remove from the oven and allow to rest for 10 mins, then spoon more glaze over the top. Can be roasted on the day or up to two days ahead and served cold.

www.ingramcontent.com/pod-product-compliance
Lightning Source LLC
Chambersburg PA
CBHW070804260726

48660CB00005B/1702